Rheumatic Healing Guide

Importance of Rheumatic Healing

By

Lennox Hubert

Copyright@2023

Table of Contents

CHAPTER 1

Introduction

Rheumatic conditions encompass a diverse array of disorders affecting the musculoskeletal system, connective tissues, and joints, presenting a formidable challenge to individuals striving for optimal health and well-being. These conditions, often chronic and multifaceted, include but are not limited to rheumatoid arthritis, osteoarthritis, lupus, and gout. As we embark on this journey of understanding and addressing these complexities, it becomes imperative to unravel the intricacies that define rheumatic ailments.

1.1 Overview of Rheumatic Conditions

At the heart of this guide lies the endeavor to provide a comprehensive overview of rheumatic conditions, demystifying their nature, causes, and manifestations. Rheumatoid arthritis, characterized by autoimmune responses targeting the synovium, contrasts with osteoarthritis, primarily a degenerative joint disease stemming from wear and tear. Lupus, a systemic autoimmune disorder, and gout, marked by the accumulation of uric acid crystals, contribute to the mosaic of rheumatic challenges individuals may face.

Diving deeper, we explore the physiological and immunological underpinnings of these conditions. Understanding the intricate interplay of genetics, environmental factors, and immune responses is crucial in comprehending the complexity of rheumatic diseases. By illuminating the distinct features of each condition, this guide aims to empower individuals with the knowledge necessary to navigate the labyrinth of rheumatic health.

1.2 Importance of Rheumatic Healing

Rheumatic healing transcends the boundaries of mere symptom alleviation; it embodies a holistic approach to restoring balance and functionality to the lives affected by these conditions. The significance of rheumatic healing lies not only in mitigating physical discomfort but also in enhancing the overall quality of life for individuals grappling with these challenges.

As rheumatic conditions often entail chronicity, the impact extends beyond the physiological realm to encompass psychological and emotional well-being. Chronic pain, joint stiffness, and the unpredictability of flare-ups can take a toll on mental health. Thus, the importance of rheumatic healing lies in fostering resilience, imparting coping strategies, and nurturing a sense of empowerment among those navigating the intricate landscape of rheumatic conditions.

The societal and economic implications of rheumatic diseases underscore the importance of effective healing strategies. By equipping individuals with the tools to manage and alleviate their symptoms, we contribute not only to personal well-being but also to a more inclusive and supportive societal framework.

In essence, the journey towards rheumatic healing is a collective endeavor, weaving together medical advancements, lifestyle modifications, and a profound understanding of individual experiences. This guide aspires to be a compass, guiding individuals and healthcare practitioners alike towards a holistic approach to rheumatic healing, where each facet of well-being is acknowledged and addressed.

CHAPTER 2

Understanding Rheumatic Conditions

2.1 Causes and Risk Factors

Peering into the intricate web of rheumatic conditions requires an exploration of the multifaceted tapestry of causes and risk factors. Unraveling the origins of these ailments involves navigating the interplay between genetic predispositions, environmental triggers, and lifestyle elements. In this section, we delve into the nuanced landscape that contributes to the onset and progression of rheumatic diseases.

Rheumatoid Arthritis:

The genesis of rheumatoid arthritis often lies in a complex interplay of genetic susceptibility and environmental triggers. Certain genetic markers increase the vulnerability to autoimmune responses, where the immune system mistakenly attacks the synovium. Environmental factors, such as infections or exposure to certain substances, can act as catalysts, initiating the inflammatory cascade. Hormonal influences and lifestyle choices may also play a role, underscoring the importance of comprehensive understanding in the quest for effective prevention and management.

Osteoarthritis:

While aging remains a prominent risk factor for osteoarthritis, it is not the sole determinant. Joint injuries, repetitive stress on specific joints, and genetic factors contribute to the breakdown of cartilage. Obesity, with its biomechanical and inflammatory implications, further amplifies the risk. Exploring the dynamic interplay of these factors provides a holistic perspective essential for devising targeted interventions aimed at preserving joint health.

Lupus:

Lupus, with its diverse manifestations, is shaped by a combination of genetic and environmental influences. Specific genetic variations may predispose individuals to lupus, and environmental triggers, such as infections, sunlight exposure, and certain medications, can provoke the onset of symptoms. Hormonal factors, particularly in women, contribute to the higher prevalence among females. Understanding these intricate connections empowers individuals to navigate potential triggers and adopt strategies for proactive management.

Gout:

Gout, often linked to dietary choices, is characterized by elevated levels of uric acid in the blood. Genetic factors can influence the body's ability to regulate uric acid, while dietary choices, particularly those rich in purines, contribute to its accumulation. Lifestyle factors such as sedentary behavior and excessive alcohol consumption further heighten the risk. By dissecting the various contributors to uric acid imbalance, individuals can tailor their lifestyles to prevent gout attacks and promote long-term joint health.

comprehending the causes and risk factors of rheumatic conditions involves peeling back the layers of genetic predisposition, environmental influences, and lifestyle choices. This nuanced understanding serves as a compass, guiding individuals towards proactive measures for prevention, informed decision-making in treatment options, and ultimately, a more empowered approach to rheumatic healing.

CHAPTER 3

Symptoms and Diagnosis

Embarking on the journey to unravel rheumatic conditions necessitates a keen awareness of the telltale signs that manifest in the intricate tapestry of symptoms. Recognizing these indicators is paramount for early intervention and effective management.

3.1 Common Symptoms

Rheumatoid Arthritis:

- **Joint Pain and Stiffness:** A hallmark of rheumatoid arthritis, joint pain is often

accompanied by morning
stiffness that persists for
extended periods.

- **Swelling and Tenderness:**
  Inflamed synovium leads to
  joint swelling and tenderness,
  particularly in the small joints
  of the hands and feet.

- **Fatigue and Weakness:**
  Systemic effects can result in
  persistent fatigue and a sense of
  overall weakness.

Osteoarthritis:

- **Joint Pain:** Osteoarthritis
  manifests as localized joint
  pain, often aggravated by
  movement and relieved by rest.

- **Joint Stiffness:** Stiffness,
  especially after periods of

inactivity, is a common symptom.

- **Decreased Range of Motion:** Gradual loss of joint flexibility and a diminished range of motion become apparent over time.

Lupus:

- **Skin Rashes:** Lupus may present with characteristic butterfly-shaped rashes across the cheeks and nose.

- **Joint Pain:** Similar to rheumatoid arthritis, lupus involves joint pain and stiffness.

- **Fatigue:** Persistent fatigue, often disproportionate to activity levels, is a frequent complaint.

Gout:

- **Intense Joint Pain:** Gout attacks are notorious for causing sudden, severe joint pain, commonly in the big toe.

- **Swelling and Redness:** Affected joints exhibit swelling, redness, and heightened warmth.

- **Limited Mobility:** During a gout attack, joint mobility is significantly impaired.

Recognizing these common symptoms forms the cornerstone of early detection and timely intervention in rheumatic conditions. It is crucial for individuals to remain vigilant, communicate effectively with healthcare providers, and undergo comprehensive assessments for an accurate diagnosis. By shedding light on these symptoms, this guide aims to empower individuals with the knowledge necessary to navigate the complex terrain of rheumatic health, fostering a proactive approach to well-being.

3.2 Diagnostic Methods

Navigating the labyrinth of rheumatic conditions demands a sophisticated approach to diagnosis, employing a diverse array of tools and techniques to unravel the complexities beneath the surface. In this section, we delve into the intricacies of diagnostic methods, where precision and thoroughness play pivotal roles in unraveling the mysteries of rheumatic diseases.

Blood Tests

Blood tests emerge as invaluable allies in the diagnostic arsenal, offering a window into the physiological intricacies that underpin rheumatic conditions. In the realm of rheumatoid arthritis, tests such as the rheumatoid factor (RF) and anti-cyclic citrullinated peptide (anti-CCP) can help identify autoimmune processes at play. Elevated levels of inflammatory markers, including C-reactive protein (CRP) and erythrocyte sedimentation rate (ESR), provide crucial insights into the intensity of inflammation in various rheumatic diseases.

Lupus, being a systemic autoimmune disorder, often leaves a distinctive footprint in the blood. Antibodies like antinuclear antibodies (ANA) and anti-double-stranded DNA (anti-dsDNA) are key players in the diagnostic landscape, unraveling the autoimmune tapestry woven within the patient's immune system. For gout, blood tests revealing elevated uric acid levels serve as diagnostic beacons, guiding healthcare providers toward a more precise understanding of the underlying metabolic dynamics.

Blood tests not only serve as diagnostic tools but also contribute to ongoing disease monitoring. The dynamic nature of rheumatic conditions requires vigilant surveillance, and blood markers provide a quantitative lens through which healthcare practitioners can gauge the efficacy of interventions and adjust treatment strategies accordingly.

Imaging Tests

Imaging tests emerge as the architects sketching the structural landscapes of joints and tissues, unraveling the silent narratives concealed within. *X-rays* stand as stalwarts in the assessment of osteoarthritis, capturing the gradual erosion of joint cartilage and the formation of osteophytes. Magnetic Resonance Imaging (MRI) delves deeper, offering a detailed panorama of soft tissues, aiding in the diagnosis of conditions like rheumatoid arthritis by highlighting synovial inflammation and joint damage.

In the quest to decipher the enigmatic nuances of lupus, imaging techniques such as computed tomography (CT) scans and ultrasound play crucial roles. These modalities unveil the impact of lupus on organs and tissues, providing a comprehensive understanding of the disease's systemic nature. In gout, ultrasound serves as a diagnostic detective, detecting the presence of uric acid crystals in joints, aiding in swift and accurate diagnosis.

The realm of imaging is not confined to diagnosis alone; it extends its reach into treatment planning and ongoing monitoring. By providing a visual roadmap, imaging tests empower healthcare providers to tailor interventions to the specific needs of each individual, ensuring a targeted and effective approach to rheumatic healing.

Clinical Examination

The artistry of clinical examination unfolds as a tactile exploration, where healthcare providers engage in a nuanced dialogue with the patient's body, unraveling the subtle nuances of rheumatic conditions. Palpation of joints reveals tenderness, swelling, and warmth, offering vital clues in the diagnosis of rheumatoid arthritis and lupus. Range of motion assessments becomes the choreography of clinical examination, unmasking the impact of osteoarthritis on joint flexibility.

Beyond joints, the clinical examination extends its gaze to other manifestations of rheumatic diseases. Skin rashes characteristic of lupus become the canvas upon which the practitioner deciphers the disease's external expression. The joint redness and swelling of a gout attack tell a visceral story that complements the laboratory findings, contributing to a holistic diagnosis.

Clinical examination, with its amalgamation of art and science, serves as the frontline in the diagnostic odyssey. It bridges the gap between the subjective experiences of the patient and the objective measures provided by blood tests and imaging studies. The patient's narrative intertwines with the clinical findings, forming a comprehensive tableau that guides healthcare providers toward accurate diagnoses and personalized treatment plans.

The diagnostic methods encompassed within blood tests, imaging tests, and clinical examination converge as a symphony, harmonizing objective data with the subjective experiences of individuals grappling with rheumatic conditions. This holistic approach transcends the confines of diagnosis, laying the foundation for a tailored and empathetic journey towards rheumatic healing.

CHAPTER 4

Treatment Options

Embarking on the path of rheumatic healing involves a multifaceted approach, with treatment options ranging from pharmacological interventions to lifestyle modifications. In this section, we unravel the pharmacological cornerstones, delving into the diverse array of medications that form the backbone of rheumatic disease management.

4.1 Medications

Medications emerge as potent allies in the quest to alleviate symptoms, curb inflammation, and preserve joint function. The pharmacological arsenal encompasses various classes of drugs, each tailored to address specific facets of rheumatic conditions.

Anti-Inflammatory Drugs

Anti-inflammatory drugs stand as frontline warriors in the battle against the persistent inflammation characterizing many rheumatic diseases. Nonsteroidal Anti-Inflammatory Drugs (NSAIDs), including ibuprofen and naproxen, provide symptomatic relief by curbing pain and inflammation. These medications are instrumental in managing the day-to-day challenges posed by conditions such as rheumatoid arthritis and osteoarthritis.

Corticosteroids, another potent class of anti-inflammatory agents, may be administered orally, intravenously, or through joint injections. While effective in swiftly alleviating inflammation, their long-term use is often tempered by potential side effects, necessitating a nuanced approach in their prescription.

Disease-Modifying Antirheumatic Drugs (DMARDs)

Beyond symptom management, the quest for rheumatic healing often involves addressing the underlying processes driving disease progression. *Disease-Modifying Antirheumatic Drugs (DMARDs)* step into this pivotal role, aiming to modulate the immune system and impede the relentless march of autoimmune responses.

In rheumatoid arthritis, DMARDs such as methotrexate, hydroxychloroquine, and biologics like tumor necrosis factor (TNF) inhibitors have revolutionized treatment paradigms. These medications not only alleviate symptoms but also strive to preserve joint integrity and function, offering individuals a pathway towards long-term well-being.

Pain Relievers

Pain relievers, while not addressing the underlying disease mechanisms, play a crucial role in enhancing the quality of life for individuals grappling with rheumatic conditions. Acetaminophen provides a gentler alternative for pain management, particularly in osteoarthritis, with its focus on mitigating discomfort rather than suppressing inflammation.

In gout, colchicine serves as both a preventive and treatment measure, alleviating pain and inflammation during acute attacks. Pain relievers, with their diverse mechanisms of action, contribute to the holistic approach to symptom management, allowing individuals to navigate the challenges posed by rheumatic conditions with greater ease.

medications weave a pharmacological tapestry, offering relief from symptoms, arresting disease progression, and enhancing overall well-being. The selection and combination of these medications are tailored to the specific nuances of each individual's condition, underlining the personalized nature of rheumatic disease management. As we explore the pharmacological landscape, it becomes evident that these medications, when integrated into a comprehensive treatment plan, serve as beacons guiding individuals towards a more empowered and resilient journey of rheumatic healing.

4.2 Lifestyle Changes

Beyond the realm of medications, the landscape of rheumatic healing expands to embrace the transformative power of lifestyle changes. In this section, we navigate through the pivotal role of exercise, physical therapy, diet, and nutrition in sculpting a holistic approach to managing and mitigating the impact of rheumatic conditions.

Exercise and Physical Therapy

Exercise and physical therapy stand as pillars in the foundation of rheumatic health, offering a dynamic counterbalance to the challenges posed by conditions like rheumatoid arthritis, osteoarthritis, and lupus.

In rheumatoid arthritis, tailored exercise routines enhance joint flexibility, strengthen muscles, and alleviate stiffness. Engaging in low-impact activities, such as swimming or walking, becomes a therapeutic endeavor, fostering overall physical well-being. Physical therapy, guided by trained professionals, provides a structured approach to rehabilitation, addressing specific joint impairments and optimizing functional capacity.

Osteoarthritis finds a formidable adversary in targeted exercises that aim to improve joint stability and reduce pain. Strengthening the muscles surrounding affected joints becomes a cornerstone, offering a natural support system that mitigates the burden on the degenerating cartilage. Range of motion exercises and aerobic activities contribute to enhanced joint function and overall cardiovascular health.

Lupus, with its systemic implications, benefits from exercise routines that prioritize cardiovascular fitness and muscle strength. Tailoring exercises to individual capabilities is paramount, ensuring a balance between promoting well-being and avoiding excessive strain.

Integrating exercise and physical therapy into the fabric of daily life extends beyond mitigating symptoms; it becomes a transformative journey towards empowerment and resilience. By fostering an active and engaged lifestyle, individuals not only enhance their physical capabilities but also cultivate a sense of agency in the face of rheumatic challenges.

Diet and Nutrition

The adage "you are what you eat" takes on profound significance in the realm of rheumatic conditions. *Diet and nutrition* emerge as influential determinants, capable of shaping the course of diseases like gout and contributing to overall well-being.

In gout, where elevated uric acid levels play a pivotal role, dietary modifications become a linchpin in prevention and management. Limiting purine-rich foods, moderating alcohol intake, and staying hydrated contribute to maintaining uric acid balance. Additionally, incorporating anti-inflammatory foods, such as fruits, vegetables, and omega-3 fatty acids, holds promise in managing symptoms across various rheumatic conditions.

In lupus, a balanced and nutrient-rich diet becomes an ally in fortifying the immune system and managing inflammation. Antioxidant-rich foods, whole grains, and lean proteins contribute to a foundation of optimal nutrition.

The role of diet extends beyond specific conditions to the broader landscape of rheumatic health. Adopting an anti-inflammatory diet, characterized by the incorporation of foods with anti-inflammatory properties, becomes a universal principle. This includes embracing a rainbow of fruits and vegetables, incorporating omega-3 fatty acids, and minimizing processed and sugary foods.

lifestyle changes encapsulate a holistic paradigm shift, where exercise, physical therapy, diet, and nutrition converge to empower individuals on their journey of rheumatic healing. It is a tapestry woven with the threads of proactive self-care, resilience, and a profound recognition of the interconnectedness between lifestyle choices and overall well-being.

CHAPTER 5

Alternative Therapies

5.1 Acupuncture

In the pursuit of rheumatic healing, the landscape expands beyond conventional medical interventions to embrace the holistic and nuanced realm of alternative therapies. Among these, *acupuncture* stands as a centuries-old practice rooted in traditional Chinese medicine, offering a unique approach to addressing the challenges posed by rheumatic conditions.

Acupuncture involves the insertion of thin needles into specific points on the body, aiming to stimulate energy flow, or "qi," and restore balance within the body's systems. While the exact mechanisms by which acupuncture exerts its effects in rheumatic conditions are not fully understood, its potential benefits have garnered attention and intrigue within the realm of complementary and alternative medicine.

For individuals grappling with rheumatoid arthritis, acupuncture presents itself as a complementary modality that may contribute to pain relief and improved joint function. The strategic placement of needles aims to enhance circulation, reduce inflammation, and promote a sense of relaxation, offering a holistic approach to managing the complexities of this autoimmune condition.

In osteoarthritis, where joint degeneration and pain are prominent features, acupuncture becomes a gentle yet potentially effective intervention. By targeting specific acupuncture points related to joint health, this therapy may contribute to alleviating pain and improving mobility, fostering a more comprehensive strategy alongside conventional treatments.

The systemic nature of lupus invites exploration into complementary approaches to symptom management. Acupuncture, with its focus on restoring balance and harmony within the body, may offer a complementary avenue for individuals seeking relief from joint pain, fatigue, and other lupus-related symptoms.

While acupuncture is not a standalone cure for rheumatic conditions, its integration into a comprehensive treatment plan highlights the evolving landscape of holistic care. As individuals embark on their unique journeys of rheumatic healing, the exploration of alternative therapies like acupuncture adds layers to the tapestry of options, encouraging a nuanced and personalized approach to well-being. As with any complementary therapy, consultation with healthcare professionals is essential to ensure a cohesive and safe integration into the broader spectrum of rheumatic disease management.

5.2 Herbal Remedies

In the rich tapestry of alternative therapies for rheumatic conditions, *herbal remedies* emerge as a time-honored thread, woven into the fabric of traditional healing practices across cultures. These natural interventions, derived from plants and botanical sources, offer a nuanced approach to managing symptoms and promoting overall well-being.

Herbal remedies encompass a diverse array of plant-based preparations, including teas, extracts, and supplements. While research on the efficacy of herbal remedies in rheumatic conditions is ongoing, certain herbs have garnered attention for their potential benefits:

1. **Turmeric:** Known for its anti-inflammatory properties, turmeric contains curcumin, a compound with potential anti-rheumatic effects. It is often used in traditional medicine to alleviate pain and inflammation.

2. **Ginger:** Renowned for its anti-inflammatory and analgesic properties, ginger may offer

relief from joint pain and inflammation associated with rheumatic conditions.

3. **Boswellia:** Derived from the resin of the Boswellia tree, boswellia extract has been explored for its anti-inflammatory effects. It is often used in traditional medicine to address conditions like osteoarthritis.

4. **Devil's Claw:** Hailing from South Africa, devil's claw is believed to possess anti-inflammatory properties and is used in herbal remedies to manage symptoms of osteoarthritis and rheumatoid arthritis.

5. **Green Tea:** Rich in antioxidants, green tea has been

studied for its potential anti-inflammatory effects. It may contribute to overall health and well-being, serving as a soothing beverage.

While herbal remedies offer a natural and holistic approach, it is essential to approach their use with caution. The potency of herbal preparations can vary, and interactions with medications or other health conditions may occur. Consulting with healthcare professionals before incorporating herbal remedies into a treatment plan is crucial to ensure safety and efficacy.

The allure of herbal remedies lies not only in their potential therapeutic effects but also in the cultural and historical significance they hold. As individuals navigate the intricate landscape of rheumatic healing, the exploration of herbal remedies adds depth to the spectrum of complementary options, fostering a harmonious integration of traditional wisdom and modern approaches to well-being.

5.3 Massage Therapy

In the realm of alternative therapies for rheumatic conditions, *massage therapy* emerges as a soothing and hands-on approach to promoting relaxation, alleviating pain, and enhancing overall well-being. Rooted in ancient healing practices and embraced across cultures, massage therapy offers a holistic avenue for individuals navigating the challenges posed by conditions such as rheumatoid arthritis, osteoarthritis, lupus, and gout.

Massage therapy involves the manipulation of soft tissues, including muscles and joints, through various techniques. While the specific approaches may vary, the overarching goals include reducing muscle tension, improving circulation, and fostering a sense of relaxation and comfort.

Potential Benefits of Massage Therapy for Rheumatic Conditions:

1. **Pain Relief:** Massage therapy may contribute to the alleviation of pain associated with rheumatic conditions. By targeting specific muscle groups and joints, massage can help reduce muscle spasms and enhance pain management strategies.

2. **Improved Range of Motion:** For individuals grappling with the stiffness and reduced range of motion characteristic of rheumatoid arthritis and osteoarthritis, massage therapy becomes a gentle intervention. The manipulation of soft tissues may enhance flexibility and joint mobility.

3. **Stress Reduction:** The impact of rheumatic conditions extends beyond the physical realm, often contributing to stress and emotional discomfort. Massage therapy serves as a holistic modality, fostering relaxation and reducing stress levels, contributing to overall well-being.

4. **Enhanced Blood Circulation:** Improved circulation is a

hallmark of massage therapy.
By enhancing blood flow to
targeted areas, this therapy may
support the delivery of nutrients
and oxygen to tissues,
promoting healing and reducing
inflammation.

5. **Improved Sleep:** Quality sleep
   is a crucial component of
   rheumatic healing. Massage
   therapy's calming effects may
   contribute to improved sleep
   patterns, offering respite to
   individuals grappling with
   conditions like lupus or gout.

While massage therapy holds promise
in the realm of rheumatic conditions,
it is essential to approach it with
consideration and consultation with
healthcare professionals. Certain
techniques and pressure levels may
need to be adapted to suit individual

needs and conditions. Additionally, communication with the massage therapist about specific symptoms and preferences is crucial to ensure a safe and tailored experience.

As individuals embark on their unique journeys of rheumatic healing, the integration of massage therapy becomes a comforting and therapeutic element, weaving its way into the broader tapestry of holistic care.

CHAPTER 6

Coping Strategies

6.1 Psychological Support

The journey through rheumatic conditions extends beyond the physical realm, often intertwining with the intricate tapestry of emotions, resilience, and mental well-being. *Psychological support* stands as a vital pillar in the holistic approach to coping with the challenges posed by conditions such as rheumatoid arthritis, osteoarthritis, lupus, and gout.

The psychological impact of living with a chronic rheumatic condition can manifest in various ways, including stress, anxiety, depression, and a sense of uncertainty about the future. In recognition of these challenges, integrating psychological support becomes an integral aspect of comprehensive care.

Ways in Which Psychological Support Can Contribute to Rheumatic Healing:

1. **Emotional Well-being:** Coping with the physical symptoms of rheumatic conditions often involves navigating a spectrum of emotions. Psychological support offers a safe space for individuals to express and process their feelings, fostering emotional well-being and resilience.

2. **Stress Management:** Living with a chronic condition can be inherently stressful.

Psychological support equips individuals with coping mechanisms and stress management strategies, empowering them to navigate the ups and downs with greater ease.

3. **Cognitive Behavioral Therapy (CBT):** CBT is a therapeutic approach that focuses on identifying and challenging negative thought patterns. It has shown promise in helping individuals with rheumatic conditions manage pain, cope with symptoms, and improve overall quality of life.

4. **Peer Support and Support Groups:** Connecting with others who share similar experiences can be immensely beneficial. Peer support and

participation in support groups provide a sense of community, understanding, and shared wisdom, fostering a supportive network.

5. **Mindfulness and Relaxation Techniques:** Practices such as mindfulness meditation and relaxation techniques contribute to a sense of calm and centeredness. These tools can be instrumental in managing the emotional aspects of living with a chronic condition.

6. **Goal Setting and Positive Psychology:** Psychological support encourages individuals to set realistic goals, both in terms of managing their condition and enhancing overall well-being. Positive psychology principles, focusing

on strengths and positive aspects of life, play a role in fostering a resilient mindset.

Acknowledging the psychological dimensions of rheumatic conditions underscores the importance of a holistic and patient-centered approach to care. By integrating psychological support into the broader treatment plan, individuals embark on a journey that addresses not only the physical symptoms but also the emotional and mental facets of their well-being.

As individuals navigate the complexities of living with rheumatic conditions, psychological support becomes a compass, guiding them towards a more empowered and resilient stance in the face of challenges. It is a recognition of the interconnectedness between mind and body, underscoring the significance of holistic care in the pursuit of rheumatic healing.

6.2 Support Groups

In the intricate tapestry of coping with rheumatic conditions, *support groups* emerge as beacons of understanding, empathy, and shared strength. These groups, comprising individuals who navigate similar challenges, offer a communal space where experiences are shared, wisdom is exchanged, and a collective resilience is forged. Whether grappling with rheumatoid arthritis, osteoarthritis, lupus, or gout, the power of shared journeys becomes a cornerstone in the holistic approach to well-being.

Key Aspects of Support Groups in Coping with Rheumatic Conditions:

1. **Shared Understanding:**
   Support groups provide a
   unique platform where
   individuals can express their
   thoughts, concerns, and
   experiences without fear of
   judgment. The shared
   understanding within these
   groups fosters a sense of
   validation, reducing the sense
   of isolation that can accompany
   living with a chronic condition.

2. **Information Exchange:**
   Members of support groups
   often bring a wealth of diverse
   experiences and insights. The
   exchange of information,
   coping strategies, and tips for
   managing symptoms becomes a
   valuable resource for
   individuals seeking practical

guidance in their rheumatic
healing journey.

3. **Emotional Support:** Living
   with a rheumatic condition can
   evoke a range of emotions.
   Support groups offer a space
   for emotional expression,
   empathy, and encouragement.
   Sharing both the triumphs and
   the challenges creates a
   supportive environment where
   individuals feel heard and
   understood.

4. **Coping Strategies:** The
   collective wisdom within
   support groups extends to
   coping strategies that go
   beyond medical interventions.
   Members may share approaches
   to managing pain, enhancing
   daily functioning, and

navigating the emotional aspects of their conditions.

5. **Advocacy and Empowerment:** Support groups often become catalysts for advocacy and empowerment. Individuals gain a collective voice, advocating for awareness, research, and improved healthcare services for rheumatic conditions. This sense of empowerment contributes to a broader impact beyond individual experiences.

6. **Sense of Community:** The camaraderie within support groups creates a sense of community, transcending geographical boundaries. Whether meeting in person or connecting through virtual platforms, individuals in

support groups find solace in knowing that they are not alone in their journey.

7. **Education and Resources:** Support groups serve as educational hubs, providing information about the latest advancements in treatment, lifestyle management, and coping strategies. Access to resources and expert insights enhances the knowledge base of individuals, empowering them to make informed decisions about their health.

As individuals engage with support groups, they become active participants in a shared narrative of resilience and hope. The collective strength forged in these communities becomes a testament to the power of solidarity in navigating the challenges posed by rheumatic conditions.

Support groups are not just spaces for sharing stories; they are dynamic ecosystems where individuals contribute to each other's healing and growth. The bonds formed within these groups extend beyond the digital or physical meeting space, weaving threads of understanding and support into the fabric of each participant's journey toward rheumatic healing.

6.3 Adaptive Devices

Navigating the landscape of rheumatic conditions often involves adapting to the challenges posed by changes in mobility and daily functioning. *Adaptive devices* emerge as transformative tools, offering individuals the means to enhance independence, mitigate physical strain, and optimize their overall quality of life. Whether grappling with rheumatoid arthritis, osteoarthritis, lupus, or gout, the integration of adaptive devices becomes a practical and empowering facet of the holistic approach to well-being.

Key Aspects of Adaptive Devices in Coping with Rheumatic Conditions:

1. **Joint Protection and Preservation:** Adaptive devices are designed to reduce stress on affected joints and preserve joint integrity. For individuals with arthritis, ergonomic tools, splints, and braces become allies in minimizing strain during daily activities, preventing further damage to joints.

2. **Mobility Aids:** Conditions such as osteoarthritis or rheumatoid arthritis can impact mobility. Walking aids such as canes, walkers, or crutches provide essential support, enhancing stability and reducing the risk of falls. Mobility aids adapt to individual needs, offering a customized solution to navigate diverse environments.

3. **Assistive Tools for Daily Activities:** Adaptive devices extend into the realm of daily activities. Tools with ergonomic designs, such as jar openers, gripping aids, and adaptive utensils, enable individuals with reduced hand strength or joint pain to

perform tasks more
comfortably.

4. **Orthopedic Pillows and Cushions:** Sleep disturbances and discomfort are common challenges in rheumatic conditions. Orthopedic pillows and cushions provide support and alignment, promoting better sleep quality and reducing pressure on sensitive joints.

5. **Adaptive Clothing and Footwear:** Dressing and footwear can be challenging for individuals with limited mobility or joint flexibility. Adaptive clothing with features such as easy closures and soft fabrics simplifies the dressing process. Specialized footwear

accommodates changes in foot structure and provides comfort.

6. **Technology-Driven Assistive Devices:** Technological innovations contribute to adaptive solutions. Voice-activated assistants, smart home devices, and specialized computer accessories offer individuals with rheumatic conditions the ability to control their environment and access information more easily.

7. **Joint-Friendly Fitness Equipment:** Exercise is a crucial aspect of managing rheumatic conditions. Adaptive fitness equipment, such as stationary bikes with adjustable resistance and elliptical trainers with low impact, enables

individuals to engage in joint-friendly workouts.

The integration of adaptive devices is not a one-size-fits-all approach; it is a personalized journey tailored to individual needs and preferences. Occupational therapists play a crucial role in assessing specific challenges and recommending adaptive solutions that align with the unique aspects of each person's condition.

adaptive devices transcend the notion of aids; they become enablers, fostering independence and empowerment. As individuals embrace the adaptive tools that resonate with their lifestyles, they embark on a journey where each device becomes a catalyst for resilience, allowing them to navigate the complexities of rheumatic conditions with greater ease and confidence.

CHAPTER 7

Prevention and Maintenance

7.1 Joint Protection Techniques

In the intricate dance of prevention and maintenance in rheumatic conditions, *joint protection techniques* emerge as a guiding choreography. Whether facing the challenges of rheumatoid arthritis, osteoarthritis, lupus, or gout, proactive measures to safeguard joint health become essential elements in the holistic approach to well-being.

Key Joint Protection Techniques:

1. **Proper Body Mechanics:**

    - Maintain good posture during daily activities to reduce stress on joints.

    - Lift objects using the strength of your legs rather than relying on your back.

    - Avoid prolonged periods of static positions; incorporate breaks and movement.

2. **Joint-Friendly Exercises:**

    - Engage in low-impact exercises such as swimming, walking, or cycling to promote joint mobility without excessive strain.

- Include strength training to build muscle support around joints.

- Work with a physical therapist to develop a personalized exercise plan.

3. **Joint Positioning:**

- Be mindful of joint positions during activities. Opt for neutral or mid-range positions to minimize stress.

- Use ergonomic tools and adaptive devices to maintain optimal joint alignment.

4. **Weight Management:**

- Maintain a healthy
  weight to reduce the load
  on weight-bearing joints.

- Adopt a balanced diet to
  support overall well-
  being and joint health.

5. **Use of Assistive Devices:**

- Employ adaptive devices
  such as canes, walkers,
  or braces to reduce joint
  strain during activities.

- Choose footwear with
  proper support and
  cushioning to alleviate
  pressure on the feet and
  knees.

6. **Pacing and Planning:**

- Break tasks into smaller, manageable segments to avoid overexertion.

- Prioritize activities and schedule rest breaks to prevent fatigue and joint stress.

7. **Joint Protection during Sleep:**

   - Opt for a mattress and pillows that provide adequate support for the spine and joints.

   - Experiment with different sleeping positions to find the most comfortable one for your joints.

8. **Avoiding Repetitive Stress:**

- Vary tasks and avoid prolonged repetitive movements to prevent overuse injuries.

- Use ergonomic tools and modify workstations to reduce strain during activities.

9. **Temperature Management:**

- Apply heat or cold therapy as recommended by healthcare professionals to alleviate joint pain and inflammation.

- Dress appropriately for weather conditions to minimize the impact of temperature on joint stiffness.

10. **Regular Health Check-ups:**

- Schedule regular check-ups with healthcare providers to monitor joint health and address any emerging concerns.

- Communicate openly about symptoms and discuss preventive measures with your healthcare team.

Implementing these joint protection techniques requires a proactive and individualized approach. Working collaboratively with healthcare professionals, including rheumatologists, physical therapists, and occupational therapists, ensures that the strategies align with the specific needs and nuances of each individual's condition.

Joint protection techniques become a daily ritual, a mindful dance that individuals perform to preserve the harmony of their joints. By incorporating these measures into their routines, individuals embark on a journey of prevention and maintenance, cultivating resilience and nurturing the delicate balance between proactive self-care and the complexities of living with rheumatic conditions.

7.2 Regular Health Checkups

In the symphony of rheumatic health, *regular health checkups* emerge as crucial orchestrators, conducting a proactive and vigilant approach to managing conditions such as rheumatoid arthritis, osteoarthritis, lupus, and gout. These checkups serve as compass points, guiding individuals and healthcare providers in navigating the evolving landscape of rheumatic well-being.

Key Aspects of Regular Health Checkups in Rheumatic Conditions:

1. **Disease Monitoring:**

   - Regular checkups allow healthcare professionals to monitor the progression of rheumatic conditions and assess the impact on joints and overall health.

   - Disease activity, inflammation levels, and any emerging symptoms are closely scrutinized to

guide treatment
adjustments.

2. Medication Management:

- Evaluation of medication effectiveness and potential side effects is a pivotal aspect of health checkups.

- Adjustments to medication dosages or changes in treatment plans may be recommended based on the individual's response and evolving health status.

3. Joint Assessment:

- Physical examinations and imaging studies during checkups provide

insights into joint health
and any signs of
progression or
deterioration.

- Joint assessments aid in
  early detection of issues,
  allowing for timely
  interventions to preserve
  joint function.

4. **Symptom Management:**

   - Individuals have the
     opportunity to discuss
     and address any new or
     persistent symptoms
     during health checkups.

   - Healthcare providers
     work collaboratively
     with patients to tailor
     symptom management
     strategies to individual
     needs.

5. **Preventive Measures:**

- Checkups serve as occasions to discuss and implement preventive measures, including vaccinations and lifestyle modifications.

- Strategies to prevent complications or comorbidities associated with rheumatic conditions are incorporated into long-term management plans.

6. **Patient Education:**

- Health checkups provide a platform for patient education, empowering individuals with information about their conditions, treatment

options, and self-care
strategies.

- Understanding the
  importance of adherence
  to treatment plans and
  lifestyle
  recommendations is
  emphasized.

7. **Psychosocial Support:**

   - The psychosocial impact
     of living with a chronic
     condition is addressed
     during checkups.

   - Healthcare providers
     inquire about emotional
     well-being, stressors, and
     coping mechanisms,
     offering support and
     resources as needed.

8. **Collaborative Decision-Making:**

- Regular checkups facilitate collaborative decision-making between individuals and healthcare providers.

- Individuals actively participate in discussions about their treatment plans, contributing to a patient-centered and personalized approach.

7.3 Long-Term Management

The journey of rheumatic well-being unfolds across time, and *long-term management* becomes the overarching framework that sustains individuals on this path. This sustained approach involves a dynamic interplay of medical interventions, lifestyle adjustments, and ongoing self-awareness.

Key Elements of Long-Term Management in Rheumatic Conditions:

1. **Adherence to Treatment Plans:**

    - Consistent adherence to prescribed medications and treatment plans is a cornerstone of long-term management.

    - Open communication with healthcare providers about any challenges or concerns regarding medications is vital.

2. **Lifestyle Modifications:**

   - Adopting and maintaining healthy lifestyle habits, including regular exercise, a balanced diet, and stress management, contributes to overall well-being.

   - Integrating adaptive devices and joint protection techniques into daily life becomes part of the long-term strategy.

3. **Regular Monitoring and Checkups:**

   - Ongoing monitoring through regular health checkups ensures that adjustments to the

management plan are
made as needed.

- Timely identification of
changes in symptoms or
disease activity allows
for proactive
interventions.

4. **Patient Empowerment:**

- Long-term management
empowers individuals to
actively engage in their
health journey.

- Knowledge about their
conditions, treatment
options, and self-care
strategies enables
individuals to make
informed decisions.

5. **Preventive Healthcare
Measures:**

- Incorporating preventive healthcare measures, such as vaccinations and screenings for comorbidities, safeguards overall health.

- Proactive management of factors that can impact rheumatic conditions, such as maintaining a healthy weight, contributes to long-term well-being.

6. **Psychosocial Support and Coping Strategies:**

    - The psychosocial dimension remains integral to long-term management.

    - Developing and utilizing coping strategies,

engaging in support groups, and prioritizing mental well-being contribute to sustained resilience.

7. **Ongoing Education:**

   - Staying informed about advancements in rheumatology, new treatment options, and self-care practices ensures that individuals remain active participants in their long-term management.

8. **Flexibility and Adaptability:**

   - Long-term management requires a flexible and adaptable mindset.

- Adjustments to lifestyle, treatment plans, and coping strategies may be necessary as circumstances evolve.

As individuals traverse the landscape of long-term management, the journey becomes a narrative of resilience, empowerment, and ongoing self-discovery. By embracing a proactive and holistic approach, individuals with rheumatic conditions navigate the complexities of their health with a sense of agency and a steadfast commitment to well-being.

7.4 Empowering Yourself in Rheumatic Healing

In the intricate tapestry of rheumatic healing, empowerment becomes the thread that weaves resilience, self-awareness, and proactive engagement. Whether facing rheumatoid arthritis, osteoarthritis, lupus, or gout, the journey unfolds not just within the realms of medical interventions but also in the empowering choices individuals make to sculpt their well-being.

Key Elements of Empowering Yourself in Rheumatic Healing:

1. **Education and Advocacy:**

   - Arm yourself with knowledge about your specific rheumatic condition, treatment options, and lifestyle management.

   - Advocate for your needs within the healthcare system, fostering open

communication with
healthcare providers.

2. **Active Participation in Healthcare:**

- Be an active participant in your healthcare journey. Engage in discussions with healthcare providers, ask questions, and express your concerns.

- Collaborate in decision-making processes, ensuring that your preferences and values are considered.

3. **Self-Awareness and Listening to Your Body:**

- Cultivate self-awareness about your body's signals

and responses to
different activities and
treatments.

- Listen to your body,
  recognizing when rest is
  needed, and adjusting
  activities accordingly.

4. **Building a Support Network:**

- Surround yourself with a
  supportive network of
  family, friends, and peers
  who understand and
  empathize with your
  experiences.

- Engage in support groups
  to connect with others
  facing similar challenges
  and share insights.

5. **Setting Realistic Goals:**

- Establish realistic and achievable goals, both in terms of symptom management and overall well-being.

- Celebrate small victories and milestones, recognizing the progress made on your healing journey.

6. **Proactive Lifestyle Choices:**

- Embrace lifestyle choices that contribute to your well-being, including regular exercise, a balanced diet, and stress management.

- Make informed decisions about adaptive devices and assistive tools that enhance your daily life.

7. **Mind-Body Connection:**

- Explore mind-body practices such as meditation, mindfulness, or yoga to foster a harmonious connection between your mental and physical well-being.

- Recognize the impact of stress on your symptoms and incorporate relaxation techniques into your routine.

8. **Advocating for Mental Well-Being:**

- Prioritize your mental well-being alongside physical health. Seek professional support if needed.

- Incorporate activities that bring joy, relaxation, and fulfillment into your life.

9. **Celebrating Resilience:**

    - Acknowledge and celebrate your resilience in navigating the challenges posed by rheumatic conditions.

    - Reflect on your journey, recognizing the strength and adaptability you've developed.

10. **Continuous Learning and Adaptability:**

    - Embrace a mindset of continuous learning and adaptability.

    - Stay informed about advancements in

rheumatology and explore new strategies for symptom management.

Empowering yourself in rheumatic healing is a dynamic and evolving process. It involves not just facing challenges head-on but also embracing the opportunities for growth and self-discovery that arise along the way. By actively participating in your healing journey, you become the author of your narrative, sculpting a story of resilience, empowerment, and well-being in the intricate tapestry of rheumatic healing.

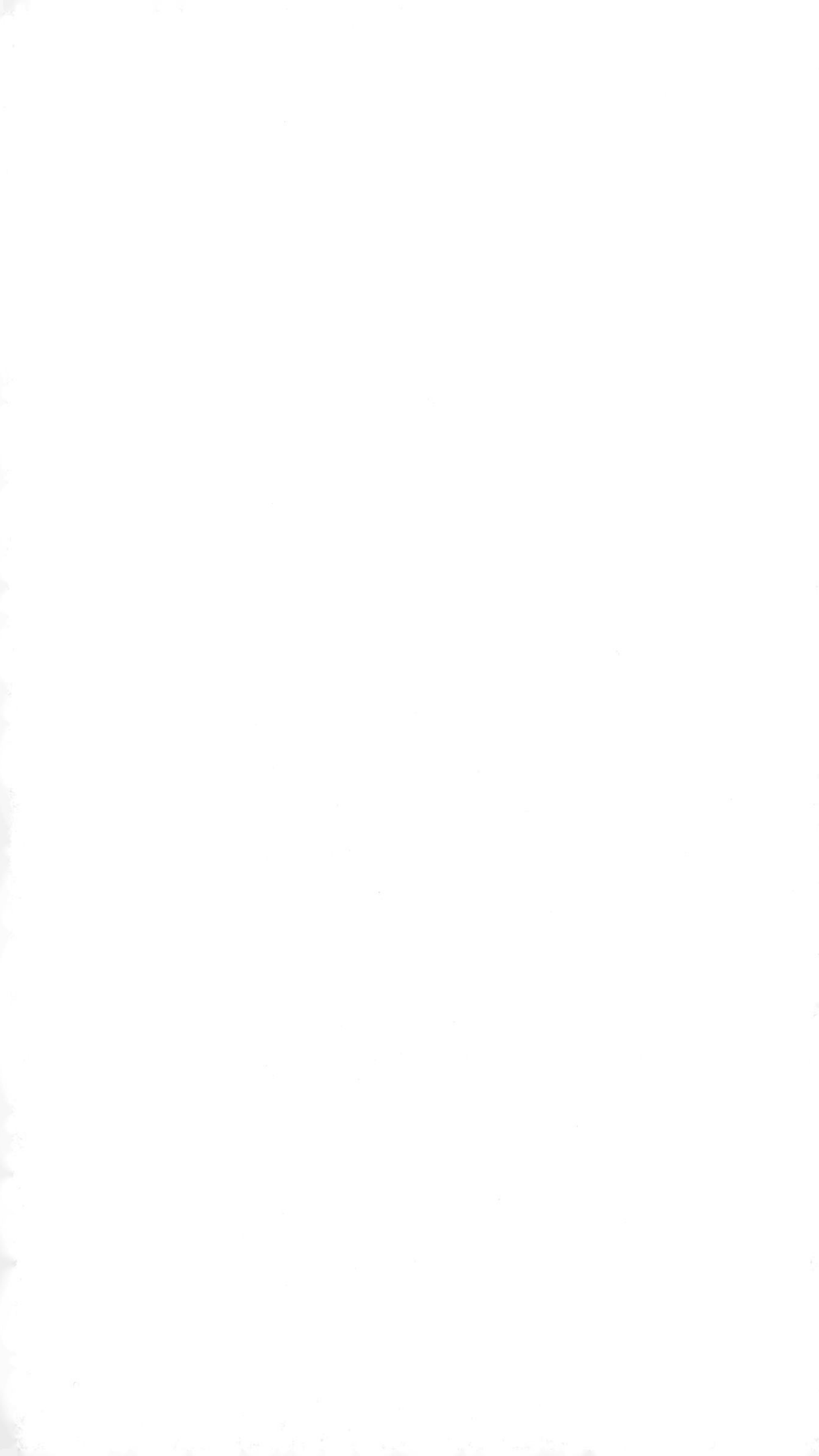

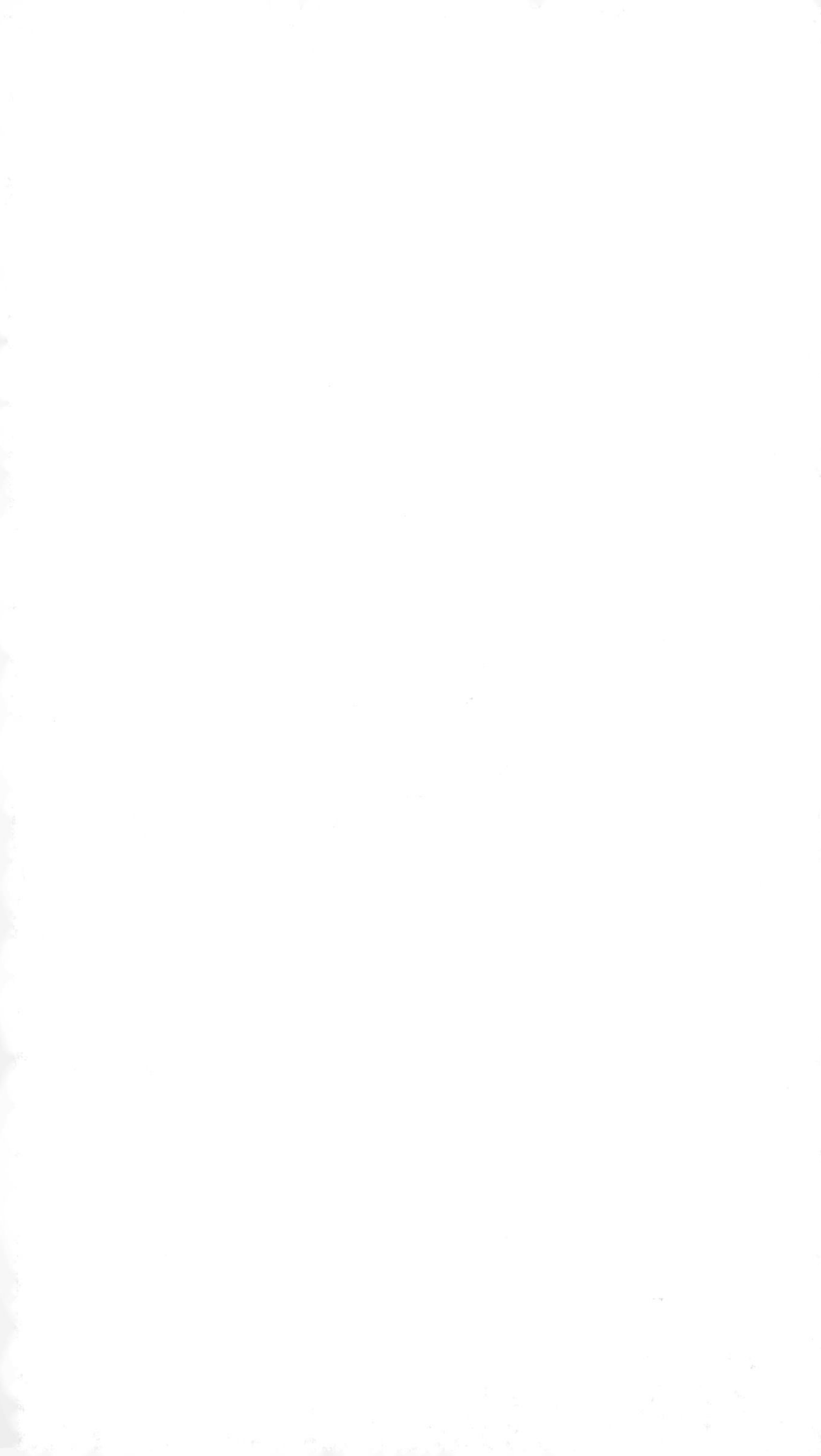

9 798867 166601